Personal Daily Log with Interactive Web-Sites

WADSWORTH
THOMSON LEARNING™

Australia • Canada • Mexico • Singapore • Spain • United Kingdom • United States

Printed in the United States of America

7 04 03 02

ISBN 0-534-58216-8

For more information, contact
Wadsworth/Thomson Learning
10 Davis Drive
Belmont, CA 94002-3098
USA

For more information about our products, contact us: Thomson Learning Academic Resource Center
1-800-423-0563
http://www.wadsworth.com

International Headquarters
Thomson Learning
International Division
290 Harbor Drive, 2nd Floor
Stamford, CT 06902-7477
USA

UK/Europe/Middle East/South Africa
Thomson Learning
Berkshire House
168-173 High Holborn
London WC1V 7AA
United Kingdom

Asia
Thomson Learning
60 Albert Complex, #15-01
Singapore 189969

Canada
Nelson Thomson Learning
1120 Birchmount Road
Toronto, Ontario M1K 5G4
Canada

Personal DAILY Log

What's in your Personal Daily Log

Exercise Pyramid

Achieving Test Success
- Effective Preparation
- Stress Relief
- Time Management
- Goal Setting

Personal Achievements

Body Composition Record Form

Body Mass Index Chart

Calories Spent During Various Activities

Warming Up and Stretching

Cardiorespiratory Exercise Record Forms

Strength Training Record Forms

Daily Nutrition Diary Forms

Get Connected

http://health.wadsworth.com

for textbook resources and more than

500 health, fitness and wellness links

Achieving Test Success:
Effective Preparation

Mastering a subject is more than simply reading and remembering the material. You must understand the material and know how to apply that knowledge.

- **Organization is the key.** Prepare yourself mentally for the task at hand.
- **Develop a schedule, and stick to it.** Be realistic in what you plan to accomplish. This will help you stay focused.
- **Get enough rest and sleep.** This can be difficult, but it is necessary to keep you alert.
- **Eat right!** You've heard it many times, and it's true. Food is energy and energy is what you need to study hard and stay healthy.
- **Exercise regularly.** The benefits are numerous. You'll think more clearly, feel better, and relieve stress that could prevent you from performing at your highest level.
- **Find a comfortable work space.** If you're physically uncomfortable, you can't expect your study time to be as effective.
- **Drink water.** You will stay alert, and you'll feel more refreshed than if you gulped a cup of coffee.
- **Familiarize yourself with the testing room.** Go to the classroom and study there.
- **Manage your stress.** Read the stress chapter in your text. Find effective ways you can control the stress in your life, rather than let it control you.
- **Take breaks.** A few minutes of relaxation can help you absorb material more thoroughly.
- **<u>Reward yourself, you deserve it!</u>**

Stress Relief

How Not to Stress Over a Test

Studies show that stress at test time can contribute to negative performance, even short-term memory loss. To avoid getting stressed when the pressure is on, take steps to avoid the possibility for stress to take hold. Here are some helpful tips.

- **Plan ahead.** A month before finals, map out a study schedule for each course. Set aside a small amount of time every day to review the course materials.
- **Be Positive.** Don't dwell on past failures, focus on how well you will do when you are prepared and confident.
- **Take regular breaks.** Get up from your desk, breathe deeply, stretch, and visualize a pleasant scene. You'll feel more refreshed than you would if you chugged another cup of coffee.
- **Study in groups as well as by yourself.** Other classmates may remember important information you may have missed. Also, talking with others about the material will help reinforce it in your mind.
- **Sweat away stress.** Even when your schedule gets jammed, carve out 30 minutes several times a week to walk, swim, bicycle, jog, or work out at the gym.
- **Cultivate hobbies.** Pursuing a personal pleasure can distract you from the stressors in your life and help you relax.
- **Master a form of relaxation.** Whether you choose meditation, yoga, mindfulness, or another technique, practice it regularly.
- **Stay in touch with close friends.** Support from someone you trust can help you put things in perspective.

Time Management

Your schedule is your business

Managing your time goes hand in hand with studying and exercising. This involves setting scheduled goals and sticking to them as closely as you can. These tips can help.

- **Tackle one thing at a time.** If you have a long list of things to do, move through the list calmly, one item at a time. Don't move on to the next item until you've finished the previous one.
- **Set realistic goals.** Separate long-term goals into smaller, more manageable ones.
- **Don't try to do everything yourself.** Ask others for help.
- **"Rehearse" a difficult task mentally first.** You'll approach it with less stress and apprehension if you have something concrete in mind. Visualize yourself achieving success.
- **Take your time seriously.** Make the most of small periods of quieter time during the day to accomplish short tasks.
- **Stay flexible and plan for disruptions.** Never schedule anything so tightly that something unexpected will disrupt everything.
- **Protect yourself against boredom.** Set a realistic goal, then work towards it consistently. Varying tasks and surroundings help to prevent boredom.

Goal Setting

Goals are critical to initiate change. Goals motivate behavioral change and provide a plan of action. Goals are most effective when they are:

1. well planned — *don't set hasty goals*
2. realistic and specific — *avoid generalities*
3. written out— *a great reference and reminder*
4. time-specific — *set deadlines and stick to them*

Personal Achievements

Goal	Date Attained

Body Composition Record Form

Goal: ____

____

Pre Test

1. Skinfolds

Men	**Women**
Chest __________	Triceps __________
Abdomen __________	Suprailium __________
Thigh __________	Thigh __________

2. Girth Measurements

Men (use inches)	**Women** (use cm)
Waist __________	Upper arm __________
Wrist __________	Hip __________
	Wrist __________

3. Other technique

   Indicate percent body fat __________

Post Test

1. Skinfolds

Men	**Women**
Chest __________	Triceps __________
Abdomen __________	Suprailium __________
Thigh __________	Thigh __________

2. Girth Measurements

Men (use inches)	**Women** (use cm)
Waist __________	Upper arm __________
Wrist __________	Hip __________
	Wrist __________

3. Other technique

   Indicate percent body fat __________

Body Mass Index

A wide range of weights is compatible with good health. Within this range, the definition of desirable or healthful weight is up to the individual, depending on such factors as family history, occupation, physical and recreational activities, and personal preferences. To determine if your weight is a healthful weight for you:

1. Calculate your body mass index (BMI). Find your height and weight in the chart on the opposite page. Your BMI is at the top of the column that contains your weight. Record your BMI here.

   ____

2. Determine if your fat distribution is associated with health risks. Measure your waist circumference by placing a tape measure around your waist just above your belly button. Record your waist in inches here:

   ____

3. Is your weight affecting your health? Do you have any of these weight-related health problems or risk factors?
   - Heart Disease
   - Type 2 Diabetes
   - High Blood Pressure
   - High LDL cholesterol
   - Low HDL cholesterol
   - Cigarette smoking
   - Osteoarthritis
   - Recurrent gallstones
   - Sleep disturbances

4. How does your current weight measure up to these considerations?
   - If your BMI is acceptable for good health and if your waist measurement is not high, you will want to maintain this weight. If you need to lose weight or gain weight, make sure you do so in a healthy way.
   - You should consider losing weight if:
     Your BMI is 30 or greater.
     Your BMI is 25 to 29 *and* you have two or more weight-related problems or risk factors.
     Your waist circumference exceeds 40 inches (for men) or 35 inches (for women) *and* you have two or more weight-related health problems or risk factors.
   - Weight loss is optional for you if your BMI is 25 to 29 and you do *not* have two or more weight-related health problems (particularly if your BMI is under 27 or you have large muscles and bones).

Body Mass Index (BMI)

Height	19	20	21	22	23	24	25	26	27	28	29	30	35	40
	Body Weight (pounds)													
5'0"	97	102	107	112	118	123	128	133	138	143	148	153	179	204
5'1"	100	106	111	116	122	127	132	137	143	148	153	158	185	211
5'2"	104	109	115	120	126	131	136	142	147	153	158	164	191	218
5'3"	107	113	118	124	130	135	141	146	152	158	163	169	197	225
5'4"	110	116	122	128	134	140	145	151	157	163	163	174	204	232
5'5"	114	120	126	132	138	144	150	156	162	168	174	180	210	240
5'6"	118	124	130	136	142	148	155	161	167	173	179	186	216	247
5'7"	121	127	134	140	146	153	159	166	172	178	185	191	223	247
5'8"	125	131	138	144	151	158	164	171	177	184	190	197	230	262
5'9"	128	135	142	149	155	162	169	176	182	189	196	203	236	270
5'10"	132	139	146	153	160	167	174	181	188	195	202	207	243	278
5'11"	136	143	150	157	165	172	179	186	193	200	208	215	250	286
6'0"	140	147	154	162	169	177	184	191	199	206	213	221	258	294
6'1"	144	151	159	166	174	182	189	197	204	212	219	227	265	302
6'2"	148	155	163	171	179	186	194	202	210	218	225	253	272	311
	Healthy Weight						Overweight					Obese		

Calories Spent During Various Activities

To calculate the exercise calories you expend per hour, find your exercise in the left column and your weight in the right column. In the place where they intersect is the figure indicating the calories burned *per hour*.

Weight (in pounds)	**110**	**125**	**150**	**175**	**200**
Exercise			**Calories expended per hour**		
Aerobic Dancing	250	285	340	395	450
Baseball	225	255	305	360	410
Basketball	415	470	565	660	750
Calisthentics (vigorous)	225	255	305	360	410
Cross Country skiing	595	675	810	945	1080
Cycling					
outdoor (5.5 mph)	195	220	260	305	350
outdoor (9.4 mph)	300	340	410	475	545
Hiking 4 mph, 20-lb. pack	355	405	490	570	650
Roller Blading	275	300	350	390	425
Rowing (sculling or machine)	620	705	845	990	1130
Running (Jogging)					
8 min/mile (7.5 mph)	625	710	850	990	1135
9 min/mile (6.5 mph)	580	660	790	920	1050
10 min/mile (6 mph)	535	605	730	850	970
Scuba Diving	355	405	490	570	650
Softball	225	255	305	360	410
Walk/Jog Combination					
13.5 min/mile (4.5 mph)	330	375	450	525	600
Weight Training/Lifting	270	310	370	430	500

Warming Up and Stretching

A good warm-up will improve performance and reduce the risk of injury. Warm-up activities usually consist of light muscular activity and some light stretching. You can also try walking, jogging or light calisthenics.

Stretching implies movement of joints through their range of motion. Stretching increases flexibility by gently stretching the soft tissue around joints. Depending on your physical activity, you may wish to stretch prior to exercising. Stretching after exercise is also beneficial. You should stretch at least 3 times a week.

Check off as you work your daily program.

Lateral Head Tilt																			
Arm Circles																			
Side Stretch																			
Body Rotation																			
Chest Stretch																			
Shoulder Stretch																			
Shoulder Rotation																			
Quad Stretch																			
Heel Cord Stretch																			
Calf stretch																			
Sit and Reach																			

Cardiorespiratory Exercise Record Form

Month						
Date	Body Weight	Exercise Heart Rate	Type of Exercise	Distance In Miles	Time Hrs/Min	RPE*
1						
2						
3						
4						
5						
6						
7						
8						
9						
10						
11						
12						
13						
14						
15						
16						
17						
18						
19						
20						
21						
22						
23						
24						
25						
26						
27						
28						
29						
30						
31						
			Total			

* Rate of perceived exertion.

Cardiorespiratory Exercise Record Form

Month

Date	Body Weight	Exercise Heart Rate	Type of Exercise	Distance In Miles	Time Hrs/Min	RPE*
1						
2						
3						
4						
5						
6						
7						
8						
9						
10						
11						
12						
13						
14						
15						
16						
17						
18						
19						
20						
21						
22						
23						
24						
25						
26						
27						
28						
29						
30						
31						
			Total			

* Rate of perceived exertion.

Cardiorespiratory Exercise Record Form

Month						
Date	Body Weight	Exercise Heart Rate	Type of Exercise	Distance In Miles	Time Hrs/Min	RPE*
1						
2						
3						
4						
5						
6						
7						
8						
9						
10						
11						
12						
13						
14						
15						
16						
17						
18						
19						
20						
21						
22						
23						
24						
25						
26						
27						
28						
29						
30						
31						
			Total			

* Rate of perceived exertion.

Cardiorespiratory Exercise Record Form

Month						
Date	Body Weight	Exercise Heart Rate	Type of Exercise	Distance In Miles	Time Hrs/Min	RPE*
1						
2						
3						
4						
5						
6						
7						
8						
9						
10						
11						
12						
13						
14						
15						
16						
17						
18						
19						
20						
21						
22						
23						
24						
25						
26						
27						
28						
29						
30						
31						
			Total			

* Rate of perceived exertion.

Cardiorespiratory Exercise Record Form

Month

Date	Body Weight	Exercise Heart Rate	Type of Exercise	Distance In Miles	Time Hrs/Min	RPE*
1						
2						
3						
4						
5						
6						
7						
8						
9						
10						
11						
12						
13						
14						
15						
16						
17						
18						
19						
20						
21						
22						
23						
24						
25						
26						
27						
28						
29						
30						
31						
			Total			

* Rate of perceived exertion.

Strength Training Record Form

Date ⟶																					
Exercise	Set	Reps*	Res*	Set	Reps*	Res*	Set	Reps*	Res*	Set	Reps*	Res*	Set	Reps*	Res*	Set	Reps*	Res*	Set	Reps*	Res*

*Reps = Repetition; Res = Resistance

Strength Training Record Form

Date →																					
Exercise	Set	Reps*	Res*	Set	Reps*	Res*	Set	Reps*	Res*	Set	Reps*	Res*	Set	Reps*	Res*	Set	Reps*	Res*	Set	Reps*	Res*

*Reps = Repetition; Res = Resistance

Strength Training Record Form

Date →																					
Exercise	Set	Reps*	Res*	Set	Reps*	Res*	Set	Reps*	Res*	Set	Reps*	Res*	Set	Reps*	Res*	Set	Reps*	Res*	Set	Reps*	Res*

*Reps = Repetition; Res = Resistance

Strength Training Record Form

Date →																					
Exercise	Set	Reps*	Res*	Set	Reps*	Res*	Set	Reps*	Res*	Set	Reps*	Res*	Set	Reps*	Res*	Set	Reps*	Res*	Set	Reps*	Res*

*Reps = Repetition; Res = Resistance

Strength Training Record Form

Date →																					
Exercise	Set	Reps*	Res*	Set	Reps*	Res*	Set	Reps*	Res*	Set	Reps*	Res*	Set	Reps*	Res*	Set	Reps*	Res*	Set	Reps*	Res*

*Reps = Repetition; Res = Resistance

Strength Training Record Form

Date →																					
Exercise	Set	Reps*	Res*	Set	Reps*	Res*	Set	Reps*	Res*	Set	Reps*	Res*	Set	Reps*	Res*	Set	Reps*	Res*	Set	Reps*	Res*

*Reps = Repetition; Res = Resistance

Daily Nutrition Diary

Goal: ______________________________

Date	Food	Amount	Date	Food	Amount	Date	Food	Amount

Use the data from this diary to obtain your computerized nutrient analysis.

Daily Nutrition Diary

Date	Food	Amount	Date	Food	Amount	Date	Food	Amount

Use the data from this diary to obtain your computerized nutrient analysis.

Daily Nutrition Diary

Date	Food	Amount	Date	Food	Amount	Date	Food	Amount

Use the data from this diary to obtain your computerized nutrient analysis.

Daily Nutrition Diary

Date	Food	Amount	Date	Food	Amount	Date	Food	Amount

Use the data from this diary to obtain your computerized nutrient analysis.

Daily Nutrition Diary

Date	Food	Amount	Date	Food	Amount	Date	Food	Amount

Use the data from this diary to obtain your computerized nutrient analysis.

Daily Nutrition Diary

Date	Food	Amount	Date	Food	Amount	Date	Food	Amount

Use the data from this diary to obtain your computerized nutrient analysis.

Daily Nutrition Diary

Date	Food	Amount	Date	Food	Amount	Date	Food	Amount

Use the data from this diary to obtain your computerized nutrient analysis.

Daily Nutrition Diary

Date	Food	Amount	Date	Food	Amount	Date	Food	Amount

Use the data from this diary to obtain your computerized nutrient analysis.

Get Connected

How to Study

Making an A: How to Study for Tests
http://www.ed.gov/databases/ERIC_Digests/ed385613.html

Study Tips on the Net
http://www.kjsgroup.com/ddss/study-tips.htm

Assessment Sites for Personal Fitness and Wellness

All the following sites are interactive and allow you to rate yourself.

Start your own fitness program
http://www.fitnesslink.com

Fitness Profile
http://www.fitnesszone.com then click Profiles

Getting Started With An Exercise Program
http://www.gsu.edu/~wwwfit/getstart.html

Activity Calorie Calculator
http://www.primusweb.com/fitnesspartner/jumpsite/calculat.htm

Body Fat and BMI calculator
http://www.freeweightloss.com/calculator.html

Health and Fitness Home Page (with many links)
http://k2.kirtland.cc.mi.us/~balbachl/fitness.htm

Stress Management and Emotional Wellness
http://imt.net/~randolfi/StressPage.html

The Longevity Game (just how long will you live?)
http://www.northwesternmutual.com/games/longevity

http://health.wadsworth.com

With more than 500 health, fitness, and wellness links.